SO-BOQ-693

Frequently Asked Questions

all about
creatine

RAY SAHELIAN, MD, & DAVE TUTTLE

AVERY PUBLISHING GROUP

Garden City Park • New York

The information contained in this book is based upon the research and personal and professional experiences of the author. They are not intended as a substitute for consulting with your physician or other health care provider. Any attempt to diagnose and treat an illness should be done under the direction of a health care professional.

The publisher does not advocate the use of any particular health care protocol, but believes the information in this book should be available to the public. The publisher and author are not responsible for any adverse effects or consequences resulting from the use of any of the suggestions, preparations, or procedures discussed in this book. Should the reader have any questions concerning the appropriateness of any procedure or preparation mentioned, the author and the publisher strongly suggest consulting a professional health care advisor.

ISBN: 0-89529-887-2

Printed in the United States of America

10   9   8   7   6   5   4   3   2

Contents

Introduction

Many of us today suffer from at least some degree of frustration with the way that our bodies look and perform. Even those who devote time and hard work to exercise may feel that their efforts are under-rewarded or wish that they could make more rapid progress. By keeping your muscles well-nourished with creatine supplementation, you may find yourself among the ever-growing number of athletes and non-athletes alike who are enjoying significant, all-natural physical changes for the better. This book, *All About Creatine*, gives you the basic facts about creatine in an easy-to-read format. We have evaluated decades of research, reviewed hundreds of articles, treated patients, and conducted a survey of creatine users to give you all of the practical information you need to use this nutrient wisely and effectively. We think that creatine can be beneficial to adult men and women of all ages. You don't have to be an athlete to benefit from creatine.

If used properly, creatine can help you:
- become more muscular and toned,
- feel more attractive with an improved body image,
- reverse muscular wasting, which occurs with the aging process,
- increase your strength and possibly improve your endurance, and
- motivate you to start and continue an exercise program.

Creatine may also give a competitive edge to more serious athletes who are looking for natural ways to increase their strength and performance. Even a small improvement can be a deciding factor in winning a race or taking home a trophy. Bodybuilders, wrestlers, and football players also know that increased strength and greater muscle mass can help improve their chances of success.

Athletes have been taking so-called ergogenic aids for a long time. These performance enhancers can sometimes make a dramatic difference in an athlete's ability to excel and give him or her a needed advantage in today's hyper-competitive sport scene. Unfortunately, not every product that is promoted as an ergogenic aid is equally effective. Some, in fact, are useless, while others can make a significant difference in strength, muscle size, and performance. Among ergogenic aides, creatine is certainly one of the most effective.

This book contains five principal chapters. Each focuses on a specific aspect of creatine use. Chapter 1 explains what creatine is and describes who can benefit from creatine supplementation. Chapter 2 looks at how creatine works. This chapter details the various ways in which creatine improves muscle size, strength, and power. It also includes the results of a number of scientific studies that verify these advantages. Chapter 3 discusses how much creatine you should take to meet your particular objectives and notes several factors that can improve the benefits you receive from this nutrient. Chapter 4 provides the latest research about creatine and sports, and Chapter 5 describes the occasional side effects that can occur with creatine use. So much research has been published in the last few years that it can be quite a challenge to keep up with it all. In this book, we provide you with a short and concise description of the practical things that you need to know about creatine so that by the time you finish this book, you will have all of the information you need to make a decision about using this supplement.

1.

The ABCs of Creatine

When athletes discovered creatine in the early 1990s, it was widely considered to be just a sports supplement. More recently, however, doctors and researchers have discovered that you don't have to be a "jock" to take advantage of creatine's power. Sedentary and elderly people can also benefit from creatine, although the greatest improvements are found in people who exercise. This chapter looks at what creatine is and explains how it may help you to gain strength and lean muscle mass. Its therapeutic benefits for certain medical conditions are also discussed.

Q. Why is everyone talking about creatine?

A. Creatine has become the most popular muscle-building nutrient ever made available to you. Why? Because it *really* works! While other supplements touted as performance enhancers have come and gone, creatine is here to stay. Its unique ability to increase strength and lean mass in a safe and effective way has allowed millions of people to achieve and maintain an attractive, muscular physique.

Whether you're twenty or eighty, male or female, an accomplished athlete or someone who has just started an exercise program, you may want to consider using creatine.

Q. What exactly is creatine?

A. Creatine (pronounced **kree**-uh-tin) is not an herb, mineral, vitamin, hormone, or steroid. It is a nutrient that is naturally found in our bodies and in the bodies of most animals. It is made from the interaction of the three amino acids (the building blocks of protein): arginine, glycine, and methionine. Creatine helps provide the energy our muscles need to move; in particular, movements that are quick and intense in nature, including the motions involved in most sports, require creatine. Approximately 95 percent of the body's creatine supply is found in the skeletal muscles. The remaining 5 percent is scattered throughout the rest of the body, with the highest concentrations being in the heart, brain, and testes.

The human body gets most of the creatine it needs from food or dietary supplements. Creatine is easily absorbed from the intestinal tract into the bloodstream. Eventually it makes its way into the muscle cells. When dietary consumption is inadequate to meet the body's needs, a limited supply can be synthesized from the amino acids arginine, glycine, and methionine. This creatine production occurs in the liver, pancreas, and kidneys.

Q. Is creatine something new that scientists have discovered?

A. Scientists have known about creatine for a long time. It was first discovered in meat by the French scientist Chevreul in 1832. Later, in 1847, a sharp observer noticed that the meat from foxes killed in the wild had ten times as much creatine as the meat from inactive, domesticated foxes. It was concluded that creatine accumulates in muscles as a consequence of physical activity. In the early twentieth century, researchers discovered that not all of the creatine consumed by humans is excreted in the urine. This led to the recognition that creatine is, in fact, stored within the body. In 1912, researchers found that ingesting creatine can dramatically boost its presence in muscle tissue. Then, in 1927, scientists discovered creatine phosphate. This discovery eventually led to the realization that creatine is a key player in energy production within the skeletal muscles (most of the muscles in your body). Studies measuring creatine's ability to influence muscular strength and sports performance have only been completed since the early 1990s.

Q. What are the benefits for the general public?

A. Most individuals have the potential to benefit from creatine. If you want to be stronger, have more lean mass, or just feel better about your body, creatine can help. Creatine supplementation has been shown to increase muscular strength and power in a wide variety of scientific studies. While some of these studies involved trained athletes, a number of others have provided insight about creatine's advantages for the general public. It is clear from this research that you don't have to be a competitive athlete to gain strength and lean mass from creatine. Many of the studies completed to date have involved college students who were primarily focused on their studies. They often engaged in light to moderate exercise, but such exercise was more likely to be walking to class or playing an occasional game of volleyball than 100-meter dashes or swim meets.

Many people note improvements from creatine supplementation during their first week of use. Creatine pioneer Anthony Almada, M.Sc., currently an Adjunct Researcher at the University of Memphis in Tennessee, notes, "There is a change in the way your body looks and feels. Your muscles feel harder and your clothing fits differently. There is also an increase in strength and fat-free mass as well as a possible reduction in body fat over time."

Q. Does this mean that you can take a few g of creatine and turn into a modern-day Superman?

A. Hardly. While creatine is a powerful supplement, it can only do so much on its own. Your muscles will increase somewhat in size because creatine increases the amount of fluid inside your muscle cells. While a 1996 study conducted by Eric Hultman found that sedentary individuals can get effective levels of creatine into their muscle cells, the greatest retention in lean mass is achieved when individuals exercise. In order to gain substantial amounts of

muscle mass, you will need to spend a few minutes
several times a week working out with weights.
Adaptations in muscle fibers are triggered by a boost
in activity. Creatine makes longer and harder exercise possible because it increases the amount of fuel
available for muscular contraction. However, if you
don't tap this extra fuel reserve by pushing yourself
physically, you may never see an adaptation of the
muscles. If you use creatine as part of an exercise program with a balanced diet that includes adequate
protein, you will see welcome improvements in your
body composition and physical energy level.

Q. Can creatine help senior citizens?·

A. Older individuals can also benefit from creatine
supplementation. "The body's energy pathways do
not change over time," notes Dr. William Kraemer of
the Center for Sports Medicine at Pennsylvania State
University in State College, Pennsylvania. "There is
no doubt in my mind that creatine works regardless
of age." Whether you're lifting barbells or grocery
bags, creatine can help preserve your strength, help
you retain muscle mass, and probably help you
regain some of the muscle mass you had earlier in
life. It may even promote faster recovery after an
injury or illness by increasing protein synthesis.

While research in this field is still continuing, scientists know enough about creatine now to suggest that it may be of great benefit to older individuals.

Creatine can help in several ways. The more strength you possess, the greater is your ability to exercise and perform everyday tasks. Stronger muscles may prevent falls and consequent bone fractures, as well. Being more muscular can also lead to an improved sense of self-esteem and well-being. Older individuals can look and feel years younger, which may encourage them to continue on an exercise program. We know that exercising leads to stronger bones and a healthier heart. Therefore, even though creatine is not technically an anti-aging nutrient, it could indirectly lead to increases in longevity by encouraging people to exercise.

As an example of creatine's power to improve the condition of aging people, let's look at one medical study that measured the impact of creatine supplementation on seventeen patients with chronic heart disease ranging in age from forty-three to seventy. When the patients took 20 g of creatine per day for ten days, their skeletal muscle strength increased by 21 percent. Torque production, a measurement of the force exerted at a distance from the body, rose by 5 percent as well. Such improvements may enhance the potential for maintaining independent living among the chronically ill or aging.

Q. Do you have to exercise to benefit from creatine use?

A. As mentioned above, creatine can provide benefits for sedentary individuals. A study published in *Cardiovascular Research*, for example, found that creatine increased muscular strength in patients with chronic heart disease, who were clearly in no position to exercise. Another study discovered that effective levels of creatine inside the muscle fibers could be achieved even when the test subjects were told to avoid exercise during the course of the experiment. However, if you are sedentary, the gains you make will be less than those you would make if you were to exercise. You will gain some muscle volume as you increase the amount of creatine stored in your muscles because creatine increases the muscles' water content. You may also gain some strength. Nonetheless, a combined program of creatine supplementation and exercise is ideal.

Q. Does creatine have therapeutic benefits?

A. Recent research has shown that creatine provides other health benefits as well. In one investigation, researchers found that twenty-eight days of creatine use improved cholesterol levels. The level of "good" high-density lipoprotein (HDL) rose by 13 percent, while "bad" very-low-density lipoproteins (VLDL) dropped by 13 percent. A similar study found that fifty-six days of creatine supplementation produced a 6-percent reduction in total cholesterol levels in the blood. Cholesterol levels remained low for four weeks after creatine use was discontinued. The results for triglycerides (fatty acids) and VLDL were even better: levels of these blood components in the same study dropped by 23 percent after four weeks of creatine supplementation and remained 26 percent below their original levels four weeks after the test subjects were taken off creatine. Blood levels for other lipoproteins were unaffected during this experiment.

Additionally, creatine has been proved effective in treating gyrate atrophy, an eye disease character-ized by night blindness, constriction of visual fields, and myopia (nearsightedness). It is caused by low levels of an enzyme involved in the breakdown of the amino acid ornithine. Untreated, the disease can lead to total blindness in 30 to 40 years. A dosage of 1.5 g of creatine monohydrate per day for one year was shown to reduce the symptoms of this disease in nearly all patients studied. No side effects were reported other than a 10-percent weight gain, pre-sumably in lean muscle mass.

Q. Are there other diseases that creatine can help?

A. Creatine supplementation also reverses the effects of guanidinoacetate methyltransferase (GAMT) deficiency. This disease can impair the development of motor control and thought processes in infants. A report published in *Metabolism* on a twenty-two-month infant found that 4 g of creatine monohydrate per day for twenty-five months brought substantial, clinical improvement, including more controlled movements and the disappearance of several brain abnormalities. Supplementation also produced normal concentrations of creatine in the brain and body.

Finally, creatine improves strength levels and torque production in patients with mitochondrial cytopathies, a group of disorders that involve a defect in the structure of the mitochondria, which is the cell's energy factory. This condition can lead to exercise intolerance, strokes, and other symptoms. Two weeks of creatine supplementation at 10 g per day followed by a week at 4 g per day resulted in a 19 percent increase in grip strength and an 11 percent jump in a torque measurement in a study by Tarnopolsky. The scientists involved in this study concluded that creatine may help these individuals during "high-intensity activity or possibly in weaning from a ventilator in an already fatigued patient."

Q. Wasn't there some controversy about creatine?

A. "Dietary Supplement Studied in Three Wrestlers' Deaths" was the headline of an article published in the December 19, 1997 issue of *USA Today*. The alleged culprit was creatine. The article begins, "The Food and Drug Administration is investigating to see whether three deaths of college athletes since November 7th are linked to a dietary supplement billed as a muscle builder."

A serious research of these three cases, however, shows that creatine is not to blame. All three of the wrestlers died the day before their meets during crash weight-loss workouts in order to qualify for their wrestling weight categories. For example, Jeff Reese, a wrestler from the University of Michigan, was the third of the wrestlers to die within a six-week period. He was attempting to lose 12 pounds in a single day. According to the December 18 and 19, 1997 issues of the *Detroit News*, he had not eaten or drunk liquids since the day before. On December 7th, under the supervision of an assistant coach, he donned a rubber suit and rode an exercise bicycle for two to three hours in a 92-degree room before becoming ill and collapsing. Wrestlers are also known to use diuretics and laxatives to lose body fluids.

ABC's *Prime Time Live* aired a comprehensive segment on January 7, 1998, regarding these three deaths. The investigative reporting by *Prime Time Live* determined that the causes of death were excessive dehydration, hyperthermia, and weight loss, along with the possible use of diuretics and laxatives. The body temperature of one wrestler had reached 106 degrees! Creatine was not mentioned as being involved in these deaths. One of us (Dr. Sahelian) interviewed the father of Jeff Reese. Ed Reese denied that his son was taking creatine. There was no creatine found in his dorm room at school and Jeff's roommate, who was also on the wrestling team, likewise denied that Jeff was using creatine. In April of 1998, *USA Today* retracted its allegation that creatine was responsible for these deaths.

It is now clear that the combination of overzealous prompting by the coaches and the unfortunate, stubborn determination of the wrestlers to shed pounds rapidly to make their desired weight categories was the cause of death for these wrestlers.

2.

How Creatine Works

Creatine has been the subject of over fifty research studies in recent years. These studies have found the nutrient to be highly effective in increasing muscle size, boosting energy potential, and enhancing strength and power. This chapter summarizes these findings and describes creatine's mechanisms of action. It also explains why not everyone gets the same results from supplementation.

Q. Why is creatine so effective as an energy source?

A. Adenosine triphosphate, or ATP, is known as the cell's "energy currency." It is used for building new tissues, nerve transmission, cardiac contraction, digestion, gland secretions, and, of course, for muscle contraction. Every cell has its own independent supply of ATP. Since it cannot be supplied by way of the blood or other tissues, each cell must continually recycle ATP by using the raw materials available inside and outside the cell.

There are three main pathways that the body employs to produce energy and all involve the use of ATP in differing ways. One of these pathways is what's called the ATP-creatine phosphate (CP) system.

The ATP-CP system is used as the immediate source of energy for the body; the other two energy pathways take some time to "kick in". Activities such as weight training, sprinting, and powerlifting, which require rapid and immediate energy for maximal exercise, are heavily dependent on the ATP-CP system.

This system involves an exchange of energy between two molecules, ATP and CP. ATP is comprised of three phosphate molecules bonded to an adenosine molecule. When one of the three phosphate bonds in ATP is chemically broken, a great deal of energy is released. This activates specific sites on the muscle fiber, which produces a muscular contraction. After ATP loses its phosphate molecule, the remaining compound is called adenosine diphosphate (ADP). ADP combines with CP to regenerate ATP. The ATP-CP system then begins again, with ATP being broken down to ADP for energy. This process goes on constantly at the start of physical work and continues as long as there is CP available to permit the reconstruction of ATP. When your supply of creatine phosphate runs out, this energy pathway grinds to a halt.

The bottom line is that your ability to regenerate ATP partially depends on your supply of creatine. The more creatine you store in your muscle cells (up to their maximum storage capacity), the more ATP can be regenerated and the easier it is to train your muscles to their maximum potential.

Q. How does creatine increase muscle size?

A. Soon after you begin using creatine, you will feel your muscles getting larger and harder. This is due to an increase in the quantity of fluid stored inside your muscle cells. As the amount of this intracellular fluid rises, it pushes against the cell membrane and actually expands the cell's volume. The microscopic boost in mass, multiplied by millions of muscle cells, results in bigger and more shapely muscles. This process is technically known as volumization. The increase in intracellular fluid levels is also thought to stimulate the synthesis of new muscle proteins, although the definitive research study on this topic still has not been completed. Scientists think that creatine also may promote the uptake of amino acids in the two contractile proteins of the muscle fiber known as actin and myosin. These two proteins are essential to all muscle contraction. The increase in quantity and thickness of these two protein-based myofilaments would result in greater muscle mass over time.

Several studies have shown increases in lean mass. A 1995 study by Conrad Earnest and his associates at Texas Women's University, the University of Texas Southwestern Medical Center, and the Cooper Clinic in Dallas, Texas, gave eight weight-trained men 20 g of creatine per day for 28 days. The researchers noted a 3.7-pound increase in total body weight with only a 0.2-pound increase in body fat. This was a 2-percent gain in the athletes' average lean mass within 30 days. A 1995 study by Balsom and colleagues at the Karolinska Institute in Stockholm, Sweden, confirmed this trend. This study gave seven men 20 g of creatine for six days. They gained an average of 2.4 pounds in total body weight in less than a week! This latter experiment did not measure the specific amount of lean mass gained by the test subjects.

Q. How does creatine enhance strength and power?

A. Creatine increases your muscles' ability to perform physical work. By providing more fuel for continued muscle contraction, creatine lets you work out longer and more intensely. And the more work you do—whether it's lifting weights, swimming 100-meter sprints, or even carrying heavy bags of groceries—the stronger you become over time. Creatine supplementation also reduces your muscles' dependence on another energy-producing pathway called the glycolytic energy pathway. This reduction lowers lactic acid production, which permits your muscles to work for a longer period of time before fatiguing. Over time, the increased work effort stimulates the body to produce additional muscle proteins as a training adaptation, resulting in increased strength and power.

Q. Are there any studies that confirm that creatine improves strength and power?

A. Several researchers have confirmed that creatine boosts muscular strength and power. In one study, the average maximum weight that test subjects could lift on bench press with one repetition (1RM) rose by over eighteen pounds in one month. This represented a 7-percent improvement. The average number of times that the participants could lift a weight that was only 70 percent of their 1RM also rose, from eleven to fifteen. The end result was that total lifting volume increased by 43 percent in only one month. The researchers explained that "these results demonstrate the efficacy of creatine monohydrate as an ergogenic aid. The ability to perform greater muscular work, per given work task, provides a greater muscular overload that may promote an increased adaptive response in muscular structure and function."

At Pennsylvania State University, test subjects took 25 g of creatine per day for a week. They experienced a significant improvement in peak power output during five sets of jump squats, along with a significant increase in the number of repetitions they could do during five sets of bench press. They also gained an average of 3 pounds of body mass during the experiment. According to Dr. William Kraemer, who participated in the study, "creatine allows a person to become stronger and more powerful. When you fill up your muscles with creatine, they have a higher force potential. This permits you to lift heavier loads and get a positive training response regardless of your age."

Another study measured work output during four different types of exercise bouts involving the high-intensity, intermittent work required in many sports. Participants received 19 g of creatine for five days prior to the first bout and 2 g of creatine per day during the actual experiment. The researchers found that creatine doubled the amount of work that could be performed during repeated bouts involving 10 seconds of work followed by 20 seconds of rest. In fact, total work rose by 62 percent for a bout with 20 seconds of work and 40 seconds of rest and by 61 percent for a bout with 60 seconds of work and 120 seconds of rest. When the participants performed all four bouts without a rest period, work output increased by 24 percent. The researchers concluded that creatine's ability to boost ATP resynthesis and reduce lactic acid concentrations permitted the additional work to be performed.

Yet another study, conducted at the University of Nottingham Medical School in England, gave 20 g of creatine to fourteen young men for five days. They then performed three 30-second bouts of maximal cycling with four-minute rest periods in between. Creatine supplementation boosted mean power output (the average amount of work accomplished per unit of time) by 6 percent, with the improvement concentrated in the first and second bouts of the routine.

Q. Does creatine improve endurance?

A. That depends on your perspective. Endurance is defined as the ability to last or continue. Creatine can help in some instances by increasing the resynthesis of ATP, which allows the body to remain in the ATP-CP energy pathway for a longer period of time. This energy source keeps the body from entering a second pathway, known as glycolysis, as soon as it otherwise would.

During glycolysis, energy is produced by the metabolism of glucose or glycogen (the stored form of glucose). The breakdown of these molecules results in the production of lactic acid, which is one cause of the "burning" sensation you feel towards the end of an exercise. Increased acidity inactivates some of the enzymes used in glycolysis, which reduces the ability of the muscles to contract. Fatigue sets in eventually and muscle movement must stop. Athletes sometimes call this "hitting the wall."

In addition to delaying the point at which the body resorts to the glycolytic pathway, creatine actually delays the point at which glycolic acidity reaches a critical level. Creatine phosphate increases the muscle's buffering capacity; it helps the individual cell to resist changes in acidity. Were it not for creatine phosphate, the glycolytic energy pathway would stop even sooner than it does. A greater supply of creatine phosphate due to creatine supplementation can assist your muscle cells as a buffer for a longer period of time. This allows you to perform more physical work and improve your sports performance in certain instances. For example, a 1995 study by Balsom and associates at the Karolinska Institute discovered that creatine supplementation resulted in an 18 percent drop in the level of lactic acid in the muscles after a ten-second, maximum-intensity workout on a cycle ergometer (a type of stationary bicycle). The amount of work performed was increased by 5 percent.

However, creatine will not help you in long-distance "endurance" events such as a marathon or in races longer than 500 meters. Such exercise is significantly fueled by glycolysis and a third energy system known as the aerobic pathway. These pathways do not use creatine.

Q. Does everyone get the same results?

A. No. Some people get more benefit more than others from creatine supplementation. This is because there is a limit to the concentration of creatine that your muscle cells can bear. The closer you are to this maximum to start with, the less improvement you will see in your strength and sports performance. Vegetarians, who are usually most deficient in creatine, tend to get greater gains than do meat eaters. Also, Paul Greenhaff reported in the *British Journal of Sports Medicine* that 20 to 30 percent of individuals do not respond to a standard creatine loading phase, where a response is defined as an increase of at least 8 percent in total muscle creatine concentrations. Currently, it is not known why some people are non-responders.

3.

Who Should Take Creatine and How Much Should Be Taken

One of the most common questions we are asked during lectures and media interviews is the correct dosage and frequency of creatine supplementation. This chapter will provide you with practical guidelines on proper dosages and explain how you can maximize your absorption and utilization of this nutrient.

Q. How much creatine is in the body?

A. The amount of creatine you have in your body depends mostly on the amount of muscle you have. (There is no creatine in body fat.) The average 155-

pound person has a total of about 4 ounces (120 g) of creatine in his or her body at any one time. Pound for pound, women may have somewhat more creatine than men. Vegetarians, for the most part, have lower creatine levels than meat eaters. The average sedentary person consumes about 2 g of creatine per day. Athletes use much more than 2 g per day, with the exact amount depending on their muscle mass, type of sport, and intensity level.

Q. Which foods contain creatine?

A. One way to get part of the creatine you need is to consume meat. Just as human muscle contains creatine, so does the muscle of most mammals and fish. As you can see in the following table, the amount of creatine in most meats is relatively constant, staying within a narrow range of 4 to 5 g per 2.2 pounds. Cod has a lower amount because of its high water content. Tiny amounts are found in milk and even cranberries. While it seems logical that chicken and turkey also contain creatine, the precise quantity of this nutrient in these meats has not yet been determined.

Foods Containing Creatine

Food	Creatine Content (g/kg)
Meats and Fishes	
Beef	4.5
Chicken	Not Available
Cod	3.0
Herring	6.5
Pork	5.0
Salmon	4.5
Tuna	4.0
Turkey	Not Available
Other Sources	
Cranberries	0.02
Milk	0.1

Q. Can I get enough creatine from my diet?

A. The average person consumes about 1 g of creatine per day. Cooking destroys some of the creatine that naturally exists in meat. While you could get part of the creatine you need from protein sources, you shouldn't dramatically increase your meat and fish consumption in order to pump your muscles full of this nutrient.

Cholesterol, which meat contains, has been linked to hardening of the arteries (atherosclerosis) when ingested in excessive amounts. Also, most meats, especially beef and pork, contain high quantities of saturated fats. For example, 2.2 pounds of raw round steak contains only 4 g of creatine, but has 120 g of fat. Porterhouse steak has a bit less creatine, but contains 325 g of fat for the same quantity! You won't live to see your nineties if you clog your arteries from the amount of meat you would need to dramatically improve your strength and power. Moreover, a high fat content in the food you eat will dramatically increase the total number of calories you consume each day. Unless your exercise intensity and frequency increase at the same rate, you will wind up gaining unwanted pounds of body fat. A far better solution is to use creatine monohydrate, which has neither fat nor cholesterol.

Q. What is a loading phase?

A. The concept of a loading phase came from scientific studies done in the early 1990s. Researchers found that a low daily dose of creatine monohydrate (1 g) produced only modest increases in the blood level of creatine and no appreciable increase in muscle mass. On the other hand, 5 g given four to six times per day resulted in a sustained rise in blood levels and a significant accumulation of creatine in muscle fibers. Therefore it was thought that higher creatine levels in muscle could only be achieved if there were a consistent elevation in the amount of creatine in the blood stream over a prolonged period of time.

The question then became how long this loading period has to be. It turned out not to be very long at all. Harris gave his study subjects 30 g of creatine per day, which, by today's standards, is a very high dose even for the loading phase. Study participants weighed around 175 pounds and engaged in only light exercise during the course of the study. Harris found that the muscles could absorb only so much creatine. After the maximum level had been reached, the excess amount was converted into a waste product called creatinine and excreted in the urine. On the first day of supplementation, 40 percent of the administered dose was excreted. This amount rose to 61 percent on the second day and 68 percent on the third day. By day three, two-thirds of the creatine consumed was wasted!

Q. What is a maintenance phase?

A. The maintenance phase is the period of time after your loading phase. Once you have filled your muscles with creatine to their maximum capacity, you only need to consume enough creatine to keep them full at all times. Lowering your dosage to a maintenance level will allow you all of the benefits of creatine supplementation.

An unpublished study shows the effectiveness of the loading and maintenance concept. In this study, subjects received 0.3 g of creatine per 2.2 pounds of body weight every day for six days. (For a 155-pound person, this would be 21 g per day.) This dosage produced a significant increase in total creatine levels in skeletal muscle. Creatinine excretion was not measured. After this loading phase, the amount of creatine was reduced to 0.03 g per day per 2.2 pounds of body weight, which is roughly equal to 2 g per day for a 155-pound person. On this low dose, muscle creatine levels were maintained at the high level originally brought about by the loading phase. Unfortunately, this study did not reveal how much the participants exercised or if they exercised at all. Nevertheless, this study indicated that high loading dosages of creatine do not need to be continued over a long period of time. To continue to take high doses of creatine after your muscles have been loaded is to waste the nutrient. Also, there is a possibility that excessive doses of creatine could place stress on some of your organs, such as your liver and kidneys, over the long term.

Although a loading phase can provide you with quicker and more noticeable gains within days of use, it is not necessary if you are willing to be patient. Some researchers have found that in sedentary individuals a dosage of 3 g per day for a month was as effective at raising tissue levels of creatine as a 20-g, six-day loading phase followed by 2 g per day for the rest of the month. We recommend that most users skip the loading phase and start with the maintenance dose in order to reduce possible side effects.

Q. What determines how much creatine athletes should take?

A. The amount of creatine that athletes should take is based on two principal factors. First, the total amount of creatine storage capacity in your body is directly related to your muscle mass. Ninety-five percent of the body's creatine is found in skeletal muscles. The more muscle you have, the greater is the quantity of storage space available and the more creatine you need to fill up your muscles.

Second, the amount of creatine you need depends on your exercise program. While a sedentary 155-pound person uses 2 g of creatine each day, rates of creatine metabolism for active individuals are much higher. If you are physically active, you will be "burning" part of your creatine dosage every day. The amount consumed, of course, depends on the workout level of your exercise routine, which is a combination of your workout's length, intensity, and frequency.

Tailoring your creatine intake to your muscle mass and exercise intensity will allow you to get the maximum gains from this powerful nutrient.

Q. About how much creatine should athletes take?

A. We recommend a loading phase only for athletes eager to bulk up quickly. The total daily dosage during this phase should be from 10 to 20 g, depending on your body weight and exercise intensity. This loading dose should be divided into two to four servings. Servings should not be greater than 5 g because larger doses, in some instances, can produce nausea, weakness, dizziness, and diarrhea. It is also advisable to drink water with each dose. The loading phase should last five days. Vegetarians may need seven days due to their generally lower initial levels of stored creatine.

After the optional loading phase, you should:

- use 4 to 10 g every day as a maintenance dose, depending on your body weight and exercise intensity,
- take one week off from creatine supplementation each month, and
- take one complete month off from creatine supplementation two times per year.

Do experiments to see which level of creatine use gives you the best results. It is because the consequences of continuous daily use for months or years are not known at present that we recommend you periodically refrain from creatine use. It's better to be cautious until more research is published on long-term creatine use.

Q. How much creatine should non-athletes take?

A. Remember, you don't have to be a competitive athlete to benefit from creatine. We think that almost everyone who wants a better-looking body can take advantage of creatine's ability to tone muscles. You should adjust the amount of creatine you take to your specific needs and desired results.

Unless you need to see immediate results, we recommend you skip the loading phase. This way, you will minimize the potential side effects of nausea or diarrhea that can occur from the high doses of creatine used for loading. The following are some general and flexible recommendations. You may:

- skip the loading phase,
- use 3 to 6 g every day or every other day as a maintenance dose, depending on your activity level,
- take one week off a month, and
- take one complete month off three times per year.

We recommend that you take these breaks because we wish to be cautious in our recommendations. Until thorough, long-term studies of continuous creatine are completed, it is best to use it conservatively.

Q. How much creatine should older people take?

A. We believe that a great, untapped potential for creatine exists in middle-aged individuals and the elderly. One of the frustrations of aging is that our muscles gradually start to shrink. It becomes increasingly difficult to regain the bulk we once had.

Putting in a lot of hours at the gym, going on long walks or runs, and playing a long tennis match don't seem to give the rewards they once did. The muscles just don't respond the way they used to.

Most of the studies that used high doses of creatine, such as 20 g per day, have been done with young volunteers. Until more research is done with seniors, we recommend that older individuals use lower dosages. The dosages for seniors are slightly lower than those for the non-athlete. If you have a chronic medical condition or are on medication, consult a physician before using creatine. Our advice, specifically, is that you should:

- skip the loading phase,
- use 3 to 4 g every day or every other day as a maintenance dose,
- take one week off from supplementation each month, and
- take one complete month off from supplementation three or four times per year.

Q. Is it OK for teenagers to use creatine?

A. We espouse a moderate approach when it comes to teen athletes and nutritional supplements. We think that teens should use only small amounts of creatine (in the 3- to 6-g range, daily) and for a limited period of time. For instance, a high school athlete could use creatine for a couple of months during the football season and then avoid using the supplement until training begins for the next season. This moderate approach may be satisfactory to the athlete while helping to resolve the concerns of coaches and the teenager's family.

We want to emphasize that athletes need to consume plenty of water in order to compensate for fluid losses due to sweating. This is particularly important when they do strenuous workouts in the humid summer heat, especially when wearing football gear.

Q. What is the best time of day to take creatine?

A. Creatine remains in the bloodstream for a period of one to two hours. This is the window of opportunity that the muscles have to draw creatine from the surrounding blood vessels and store it in their cells.

If you exercise, the ideal times to take creatine are right before and right after your workouts. Taking it before exercise allows the nutrient to circulate in the blood during your routine so your muscles can quickly replenish the creatine metabolized during exercise. Consuming it after your workout improves recovery and seems to help stimulate additional protein uptake and synthesis in the critical hour after you stop exercising. If you are dividing your daily maintenance dose into only two parts, take at least one of them before or after your workout. If you are loading, include these two times in your regimen. This will give your muscles several windows of opportunity throughout the day.

While these suggestions will help you to maximize gains from creatine, it's important to keep things in perspective. Creatine is not a nutrient that flushes out of your muscles in a short time. Unlike water-soluble vitamins, which cannot be stored by the body, creatine accumulates in your muscle cells. This means that the issue of timing is not very critical.

Q. Should I take creatine with carbohydrates?

A. While creatine should be consumed with at least 3 to 4 ounces of liquid, some liquids are better than others for achieving the optimal benefit. This is because the shuttle system used to transport creatine into the muscle fibers involves insulin. You want to mix your creatine with a carbohydrate source that will cause a temporary increase, or spike, in the insulin level of your blood. This increases the amount of creatine that gets transported into your muscle cells while reducing the amount that is excreted. Almost all the research studies to date have used glucose as a sugar source. A study by Green found that creatine concentrations in muscle rose an additional 36 percent on average when the study participants added nearly 100 g of simple sugars to the 5 g of creatine they consumed. One hundred grams is quite a lot of sugar, and it may not be healthy to consume this amount on a regular basis. Anecdotal evidence suggests that smaller amounts of carbohydrates are also effective.

Fruit and vegetable juices are good options. Juices contain large amounts of fructose and other simple sugars. These are assimilated relatively quickly, so they are perfectly acceptable as a creatine vehicle. However, since creatine in excessive doses can cause loose stools, the one drink we don't recommend is prune juice.

Sometimes, people have been told falsely to avoid the use of citrus juices, such as orange juice, with creatine. The reason given is that the acidity of these juices converts creatine into creatinine, which is the waste product of creatine metabolism. However, creatinine is formed in muscles, not in a glass. Moreover, the citric acid in orange and grape-fruit juices is insignificant compared to the concentrated hydrochloric acid found in the stomach. If creatine can make it through the stomach acid and into the body, orange juice certainly will not hurt.

Q. Can I take creatine with my meals?

A. Anecdotal evidence and the results of one study indicate that creatine can be consumed with meals. This is not particularly surprising because we know that the creatine contained in meat is absorbed during meals. Although the fat and protein in the meal may reduce the insulin spike achieved, the creatine is apparently still assimilated and later absorbed by the muscle cells as long as the meal contains sufficient carbohydrates, such as a baked potato, bread, rice, or pasta. Mixing your creatine with food would also minimize any gastrointestinal discomfort and is a preferred option for people with sensitive stomachs.

A recent study found significant improvements in body weight, fat-free and bone-free mass, lifting volumes, and total work performance when football players consumed creatine for four weeks during their three daily meals. These results are similar to the other creatine studies to date, which have involved creatine taken by itself on an empty stomach or combined with a simple sugar such as glucose or dextrose.

It is not yet known whether taking creatine with a meal or on an empty stomach with a carbohydrate drink is more effective. You may wish to try both options to find the one that suits you best.

Q. Does caffeine reduce the effects of creatine?

A. One study found that the benefits of creatine are counteracted when creatine is consumed with large amounts of caffeine—the equivalent of 10 cups of coffee. The study found that while caffeine did not reduce the increase in creatine phosphate levels within the muscle fibers, torque production (a measure of strength) in caffeine/creatine users was 10 to 20 percent lower than in test subjects who took creatine alone. In fact, torque production for the users of creatine with caffeine was no different from the placebo group. Based on this research, you should stay away from high-potency caffeine pills. Mixing creatine into drinks with caffeine, at least according to this study, may also reduce or even neutralize the performance-enhancing effects of this nutrient in the short term.

Q. Are there any supplements that act synergistically with creatine?

A. People have combined creatine with virtually every supplement on the market, ranging from simple protein powders to vanadyl sulfate, chromium, androstenedione, pregnenolone, dehydroepiandrosterone (DHEA), and hydroxymethylbutyrate (HMB). Unfortunately, there has been no published research on this subject to date. However, our clinical experience does not reveal any substances that definitely should be avoided while using creatine. Given the benign nature of creatine and its easy elimination from the body, this is not surprising.

We have come across anecdotal reports that the combination of creatine with natural hormones can produce better results. No scientific studies have been published regarding these combinations. Hormone supplements that could potentially help include androstenedione and DHEA, though we cannot recommend their regular use because of the numerous side effects that they have been known to cause.

Q. Should I cycle my creatine use?

A. Creatine is a natural nutrient, not a hormone. Therefore, it does not impact the body in the same way that anabolic steroids do. Nonetheless, we think that it is wise to take breaks from creatine use. We recommend this because we don't know the long-term effects of daily creatine use. Although there has been no mention in the medical literature of a person's own creatine production shutting off permanently or even temporarily as a result of creatine supplementation, it would be best to take occasional breaks in order to allow the body to make its own creatine. You could cycle creatine every other day, every other week, or follow the recommendations we have outlined earlier in this book. Since creatine is trapped within the muscle fibers for an extended period of time, such a hiatus should not produce any major creatine loss within your muscle tissues, and you should quickly regain most if not all of your muscle mass shortly after you start taking creatine again.

Q. How long does creatine stay in the body?

A. While creatine lasts only one to two hours in blood plasma, once it enters the muscle fiber it gets "trapped" there for a relatively long time. As a result, creatine concentrations within muscle are 200 times greater than they are in the blood surrounding the muscles. As mentioned, a sedentary 155-pound man metabolizes an estimated 2 g of creatine per day. Scientists recognize that turnover is greater for active persons and athletes with greater muscle mass, but no one has yet analyzed the precise turnover rate for these individuals.

Two studies have shown that creatine levels decline over the course of several weeks rather than days, so don't worry if you forget to take it for a day or two. After a month, muscle creatine levels return to normal when supplementation has been discontinued after the initial loading phase.

Q. What happens if I take too much?

A. There is an upper limit to the amount of creatine your body can store. Studies indicate that no more than 4 g of creatine can be accumulated in each kilogram of muscle tissue. Supplementation in excess of the amount required to maintain this level will either be excreted as creatine or metabolized to creatinine and then excreted in the urine. This is not only expensive, but it may place metabolic stress on your body, particularly your kidneys.

Q. What happens if I stop taking creatine?

A. Researchers have shown that creatine levels decline slowly over the course of a month when there is no additional supplementation. As your muscles gradually lose their additional creatine stores, some of the results obtained from the supplement will disappear. However, our experience indicates that muscle mass gains quickly return after you resume your creatine use after a break.

There has not been extensive research in this area; at this point estimates of muscle loss are pure conjecture. It may well be that part of the muscle mass and strength gained from creatine endures after supplementation ends. However, at this point there can be no certainty in the matter.

4.

Information for Specific Sports

Creatine may have benefits for athletes in a number of sports. Bodybuilders, powerlifters, swimmers, certain track and field athletes, and rowers improve their performance in many instances with creatine supplementation. This chapter looks at the possible benefits for men and women in some sports.

Q. What are the benefits for body-builders?

A. Bodybuilders were among the first athletes to discover creatine. Bodybuilders have two main objectives in their sport: increasing muscular size and reducing body-fat levels to permit greater definition and vascularity. Creatine helps on both counts. Virtually all bodybuilding movements are fueled by the two anaerobic energy pathways: ATP-CP and glycolysis. Since glycolysis produces lactic acid, which eventually makes the muscle fibers so acidic that muscular movement must stop, it's best to keep the body in the ATP-CP system for as long as possible. This enables the bodybuilder to achieve the greatest work output and the highest level of exercise intensity, which results in growth adaptations over time. Creatine also produces a volumization of the muscles due to greater intracellular fluid levels.

Creatine supplementation loads the muscle cells with as much raw material for ATP resynthesis as possible. It also appears to promote greater nitrogen retention and protein synthesis by increasing intracellular water and strength levels. As long as the athlete gives his or her body the other raw materials for muscle growth (such as amino acids, vitamins, and minerals) and allows himself or herself adequate time between workouts to permit full recovery from the stresses of training, the end result will be an increase in lean muscle mass.

The second objective of bodybuilding, as we have said, is to decrease body fat. Creatine also appears to lower body fat levels. About a third of the respondents to a survey we conducted mentioned reduced body fat as a benefit of creatine use. While the mechanism for this improvement is still unclear, it appears to relate to a higher energy expenditure resulting from creatine-enabled increases in training volume and total muscle mass. Also, as your muscle size increases, the surrounding fatty layer is spread over a wider area, which reduces its thickness and makes your muscles appear more defined. These gains in definition and vascularity are highly prized in bodybuilding, where competitive athletes often step on stage with body fat levels as low as 3 percent.

Q. What are the benefits for powerlifters?

A. Powerlifters train in order to lift as much weight as possible. There are three competitive events in powerlifting: bench press, deadlift, and squat. Each event requires the athlete to perform only a single repetition of a movement. This action is powered exclusively by the ATP-CP system. Powerlifters use creatine to maximize their ability to resynthesize ATP quickly and under very demanding circumstances. This intensifies their explosiveness and muscular strength. Creatine's apparent ability to enhance protein synthesis may also boost the number of myofilaments within the muscle fibers, which could lead to additional gains in muscular power over time. Furthermore, creatine-induced gain in muscle mass, while not considered as a judging criterion for this sport, may nevertheless help to "psyche out" competitors when you approach the lifting platform. However, mass increases can sometimes push you over the weight limit and into another class. As a result, size gains (and creatine dosages) may need to be tailored to your specific situation.

Q. What are the benefits for swimmers?

A. Swimmers may improve their performance with creatine as well. Several members of the U.S. swim team at the 1996 Summer Olympics reportedly used the supplement to improve their times.

A study published in the *International Journal of Sports Nutrition* found significant improvements in swimming sprint times with creatine supplementation. Eighteen male and female competitive swimmers took 21 g of creatine and 4 g of maltodextrin per day for 9 days. Compared to the control group, the creatine users had reductions of 0.27 seconds, 0.93 seconds and 0.36 seconds for the first, second, and third, 100-meter bouts, respectively. There were 60 seconds of rest between each bout. "This resulted in a cumulative gain of 3.1 meters over [the control group], enough to provide a clear competitive edge," noted Dr. Rick Kreider, one of the study's researchers. "There were also improvements of 5 percent in mean total work and average power for the three sprint tests."

Other research may indicate that a higher-dosage loading phase, as in the study above, or a higher daily dosage during the maintenance phase is necessary for swimmers to see significant results.

Q. Are there benefits for sprinters?

A. Track and field athletes were some of the earliest users of creatine. Competitive use of this supplement was reported as long ago as the 1992 Barcelona Olympics. An article in the *London Times* reported that gold-medalist Linford Christie had used creatine for his 100-meter win. Sally Gunnell, who won the gold medal in the 400-meter hurdles, was another creatine user. Since 1992, the use of creatine in this sport has increased.

Researchers have found that creatine supplementation reduced running times for athletes who performed four bouts of a 300-meter sprint with three minutes of rest in between. There was an average 1.5-second reduction in mean running time, and the most pronounced drop in time was on the final 300-meter bout. The increases in speed were even greater when the runners did four bouts of a 1,000-meter sprint with four minutes of rest in between. The mean running time dropped by a total of 13.0 seconds for the four bouts and by 5.5 seconds during the last bout alone. The test subjects had taken a total of 30 g of creatine along with 30 g of glucose per day for six days. As is often the case, some research contradicts these findings and shows little or no difference between creatine users and nonusers in this sport.

Q. What are the benefits for other track and field events?

A. Creatine may improve performance in the javelin, discus, and shot-put. These events place a high value on explosive movement, which is fueled almost exclusively by the ATP-CP energy pathway. The added strength and power that these athletes would get from creatine should theoretically allow them to throw their projectiles further and with greater consistency, particularly during repeated bouts. No studies on these events have been published to date.

Creatine may improve performance in the broad and high jumps due to increased strength and power or it may be counterproductive because of the increase in body weight. No studies are available to indicate creatine's role in these events. For longer races creatine use may not be beneficial.

Although creatine should theoretically help buffer the buildup of lactic acid which can limit performance during longer-distance events, a 1993 study by Balsom found that there was actually an average increase of 25.8 seconds in the time of a 6,000-meter run on a forest track with undulating terrain. Test subjects had consumed 20 g of creatine along with 4 g of glucose per day for six days. The researchers suggested that the average 2 pound increase in the body mass of the creatine users may have been responsible for the drop in performance. This weight gain appears to have negated the strength and buffering benefits of the supplement. The precise running distance beyond which creatine is detrimental to performance has yet to be determined.

Q. What are the benefits for rowers?

A. Only one study has been published about creatine and rowing. In it, Harry Rossiter from the University of Birmingham in England gave a group of rowers 0.25 g of creatine per 2.2 pounds of body weight (17.5 g for a 155-pound athlete) for five days and compared the results to a group receiving a placebo. Creatine supplementation improved rowing speeds by 2.3 seconds (just over 1 percent) during a 1,000-meter event. While the athletes using creatine always rowed faster than those taking the placebo, the differential between the two groups increased as the event progressed. During the final 400 meters of the race, creatine users had significantly greater speeds than those taking the placebo. Rossiter found that creatine increased the power production of these competitive rowers instead of changing their stroke rate. He attributed these improvements in part to the buffering capacity of creatine. Additional studies are needed before we can be certain about creatine's benefits for rowers.

Q. What are the advantages for wrestlers and football players?

A. Creatine could either help or hurt a wrester's performance. Creatine's ability to increase muscular strength and endurance is often cited as the biggest advantage for this sport. Clearly, if wrestlers are stronger, they are more likely to escape from holds and pin opponents. However, wrestling events require that an athlete compete within a particular weight category. The increase in body weight from additional muscle mass could push a wrestler into the next weight class, which would be a disadvantage.

Football players are not limited to a weight class. In fact, except for the quarterback and running backs, the more muscle mass the athlete has, the greater his effectiveness. Although no studies have been completed on football performance, many professional and college football players have been supplementing with this nutrient.

Q. What are the possible benefits for other sports?

A. Unfortunately, research on creatine use among athletes is still in the very early stages. So far, this nutrient has only been tested in a limited number of sports. As a rule, creatine has been found to be effective in sports that require an increase in muscle mass and strength. It is difficult for us to predict whether creatine will be helpful in sports where agility, speed, and hand-eye coordination are the primary factors that determine success. Therefore, we don't know the role that creatine will play in boxing, martial arts, tennis, basketball, baseball, volleyball, soccer, hockey, and other similar sports.

A 1996 study by Bosco, however, showed the benefits of creatine for sports that involve jumping and short bursts of running. Fourteen male athletes participated in the study, taking either 20 g of creatine with 20 g of glucose for five days or a glucose placebo. When the athletes jumped continuously for 45 seconds, the average jumping height of the creatine group rose by 7 percent, with the greatest improvement taking place during the first 30 seconds.

5.

Side Effects and Contraindications

Although creatine has proved to be the safest and most effective muscle-building supplement available over the counter, no nutrient is completely risk-free when misused. There are side effects that can occur if you take an excessive dose of this supplement. There are also certain individuals with medical conditions who should be cautious about using creatine. This chapter discusses these side effects and contraindications.

Q. All this sounds pretty good, but are there any side effects?

A. Experiments with the administration of creatine have been conducted since the early 1990s.

Although most of the participants in these studies did not experience any side effects from their creatine use, our clinical experience has been that some individuals can develop temporary side effects in certain situations. However, personal interviews with people who have used creatine for over two years do not show any long-term side effects.

We have supervised many patients and individuals who have taken creatine in varying dosages. Also, as part of our research for this book, we distributed a survey to men and women in three states.

The creatine users responding to our survey indicate that creatine can sometimes produce minor side effects if not used appropriately. None of the survey respondents reported any toxicity or side effect serious enough to make them discontinue their use of the supplement. However, a third of the men and women mentioned some temporary side effect connected with their creatine use, particularly during the optional loading phase. Bear in mind that most of these survey respondents were athletes who took relatively high doses of creatine. If you are a senior citizen or non-athlete and use the lower dosages that we recommend for your category, the probability of experiencing any side effect seems to be low.

Q. What were the most common problems reported?

A. The most common complaint was mild diarrhea during the loading phase, particularly when the serving size was greater than 8 g. Taking creatine on an empty stomach also increased the chances of getting diarrhea. Loose stools were rare when the serving size was 5 g or less. Infrequent complaints included occasional gas, flatulence, stomach cramps, dizziness, and temporary weakness. All of these conditions responded to changes in the serving size or total dosage level.

One caution worth making is that the studies that used high dosages of creatine, such as 20 g per day, were only a month or less in duration. As a result, we do not have controlled, scientific studies that indicate exactly what happens to users taking large amounts of creatine for many months or even years. The only studies that have involved long-term supplementation used dosages of 8 g or less per day. We don't fully know yet the consequences of high-dosage, long-term supplementation.

Q. Is there a connection between creatine and muscle tears and pulls?

A. Another controversy is the supposed connection between creatine and an increase in muscle pulls and tears. A small number of coaches and athletes have reported that the incidences of these problems increased with creatine use. In order to determine the correlation—if any—between creatine and muscle injury, Dr. Richard Kreider of the University of Memphis performed five double-blind, placebo-controlled studies ranging from 9 to 84 days in length. The 164 participants included off-season football players, non-competitive bodybuilders and swimmers, and elite endurance athletes. Everyone completed a detailed questionnaire about his or her experiences at the end of the study. The results were presented at the National Strength and Conditioning Association's meeting in Nashville in June 1998. "These studies show that there is no correlation between creatine and muscle injuries whatsoever," notes Dr. Kreider. "We studied a wide variety of sports and intensity levels, but creatine proved to be safe across the board."

Nonetheless, to be on the cautious side, we advise new users of creatine to increase weight and intensity levels gradually. It is important to give muscle and connective tissue time to adjust to gains in strength.

Q. Does creatine harm the kidneys?

A. One of the metabolic by-products of creatine metabolism is creatinine. It is normally collected by the kidneys and excreted along with other waste products. Creatinine levels in the blood are relatively stable in people with healthy kidneys. If creatinine levels are high, doctors suspect kidney damage.

When you supplement with creatine, sometimes there can be an increase in the creatinine levels in your blood. This is because more creatine is metabolized due to the larger amounts you are now using during your workouts. It is not a sign of illness, and the creatinine is eventually processed by the kidneys and excreted. However, you should advise your doctor that you are taking creatine so he or she does not misinterpret your blood tests and wrongly suspect that you have a kidney problem.

A recent study by Poortmans looked into the impact of short-term creatine supplementation on the kidneys. Five men took 20 g of creatine for five days. Testing revealed that there was a 3.7-fold increase in the amount of creatine in the blood and a 90-fold increase in urine, on average. Despite this high rate of creatine excretion, there was no significant increase in the amount of creatinine in the blood or urine. The researchers also found that there was no detrimental effect on kidney filtration rates and protein excretion rates. At least in the short term, creatine supplementation does not appear to "stress" the kidneys.

Q. Are there any drug interactions?

A. No studies have been done that test the interaction of creatine with pharmaceutical medicines. As you know, there are hundreds of drugs prescribed by doctors, and it is often difficult to predict the way in which these drugs will interact. Based on our knowledge of creatine and pharmaceutical medicines, we do not expect any significant interactions between creatine and hormones, antidepressants, sedatives, or analgesics. If you currently have a medical condition and are taking drugs on a regular basis, we strongly advise that you consult your physician if you are planning to supplement with this nutrient.

Q. What should I do if a side effect occurs?

A. That depends on the side effect. If you experience diarrhea or nausea, reduce the serving size to less than 5 g per serving. For most people, this eliminates the problem. If you were taking your entire creatine dose at one time during the day, try dividing it into two or even three doses. You could also try taking creatine with your meals. This often reduces the incidences of diarrhea and nausea because the creatine is blended with your food, which effectively dilutes it in your stomach and intestines. Also, be sure to drink 4 to 8 ounces of fluid with each dose. If these suggestions do not eliminate the diarrhea and nausea, you should stop using creatine.

If you experience any other side effect while using creatine, consult your doctor.

For unknown reasons, a small number of people are simply unable to use this normally benign nutrient.

Q. Are there any people who should not use creatine?

A. If you have any medical problems, we recommend that you consult a physician before supplementing with creatine. This is especially important if you have kidney or liver disorders. The kidneys are the main organs responsible for eliminating creatinine. If you have a kidney disease and take a high dose of creatine, it is possible that your blood creatinine levels could rise to unacceptable levels.

Conclusion

This book has provided you with an in-depth look at creatine. This fascinating nutrient has received an increasing amount of attention lately as scientists have discovered its true potential for boosting strength and physical performance. While some supplements have their days in the sun and then fade into the shadows, creatine is here to stay. Its benefits have been proved in controlled, scientific studies. Respected journals, including *Clinical Science*, the *Journal of Biological Chemistry*, and the *International Journal of Sports Nutrition* have published articles on creatine that show its advantages as a muscle-building nutrient.

Now, even people who had become jaded from the hype on some other supplements have become true believers. They have discovered first-hand that creatine works. Middle-aged and older individuals are finding that creatine can help them regain their muscle mass and strength. Bodybuilders and powerlifters have seen their strength and muscle mass increase. Every day, more and more people are finding that creatine can help them achieve their physical goals.

We wish you the best of luck in your training. If you're currently sedentary, we expect that the quick improvements in muscle size you get from creatine will encourage you to become more physically active. The proper use of creatine will help you look and feel your best regardless of your age.

Glossary

Adenosine triphosphate (ATP). An energy-rich compound found in every cell of the body. It is used for all of the cell's energy requirements.

Amino acids. The "building blocks" of protein synthesis. There are 20 different amino acids used by the body. They are combined in various ways to create thousands of types of proteins.

Atrophy. A reduction in muscle size due to illness, injury, or a more sedentary lifestyle.

Creatine monohydrate. A dietary supplement that has been shown to increase the levels of creatine phosphate available to muscle cells.

Creatine phosphate (CP). A molecule in the cell that serves as an energy-producing component.

Creatinine. A by-product of creatine metabolism which is excreted in the urine.

Energy pathway. One of three ways in which the body can produce energy. The energy pathway used for immediate muscle movement involves adenosine triphosphate (ATP) and creatine phosphate (CP). See also glycolysis.

Ergogenic aid. A nutritional supplement that enhances muscular strength or performance.

Glycolysis. An energy pathway that uses glucose or glycogen (the storage form of glucose) for fuel.

Metabolism. Chemical changes that take place inside the body's tissues that involve the creation of larger molecules (anabolism) or the breakdown of molecules (catabolism).

Protein synthesis. The creation of new amino acids or other proteins within the cells of the body.

Torque. A measurement of the force exerted by a muscle at a distance from the body.

Volumization. An increase in the size of a cell due to increased amounts of fluid inside the cell membrane.

References

Balsom P, Harridge S, Soderlund K, Sjodin B, Ekblom B, "Creatine supplementation per se does not enhance endurance exercise performance," *Acta Physiol Scan* 149 (1993): 521-523.

Balsom P, Soderlund K, Ekblom B, "Creatine in humans with special reference to creatine supplementation," *Sports Med* 18(4) (1994): 268-280.

Balsom P, Soderlund K, Sjodin B, Ekblom B, "Skeletal muscle metabolism during short-duration, high-intensity exercise: influence of creatine supplementation," *Acta Physiol Scan* 154 (1995): 303-310.

Birch R, Noble D, Greenhaff P, "The influence of dietary creatine supplementation on performance during repeated bouts of maximal isokinetic cycling in man," *Eur J Appl Physiol* 69 (1994): 268-270.

Bosco C, Tihanyi J, Pucspk J, Kovacs I, Gabossy A, Colli R, Pulvirenti G, Tranquilli C, Foti C, Viru M, Viru A, "Effect of oral creatine supplementation on jumping and running performance," *Int J Sports Med* 18 (1997): 367-372.

Earnest C, Almada A, Mitchell T, "High-performance capillary electrophoresis—pure creatine monohydrate reduces blood lipids in men and women," *Clin Sci 91* (1996): 113-118.

Earnest C, Snell P, Rodriguez R, Almada A, Mitchell T, "The effect of creatine monohydrate ingestion on anaerobic power indices, muscular strength and body composition," *Acta Physiol Scan 153* (1995): 207-209.

Febbraio M, Flanagan T, Snow R, Zhao S, Carey M, "Effect of creatine supplementation on intramuscular TCr, metabolism and performance during intermittent, supramaximal exercise in humans," *Acta Physiol Scan* 155(4) (1995): 387-395.

Fitch C, Shields R, Payne W, Dacus J, "Creatine metabolism in skeletal muscle: specificity of the creatine entry process," *J Biol Chem* 243(8) (1968): 2024-2027.

Gordon A, Hultman E, Kaijser L, Kristjansson S, "Creatine supplementation in chronic heart failure increases skeletal muscle creatine phosphate and muscle performance," *Cardio Res* 30 (1995): 413-418.

Green A, Hultman E, Macdonald I, Sewell D, Greenhaff P, "Carbohydrate ingestion augments skeletal muscle creatine accumulation during creatine supplementation in humans," *Am J Physiol* 271 (1996): E821-E826.

Greenhaff P, "Creatine supplementation: recent developments," *Br J Sports Med* 30 (1996): 276-281.

Greenhaff P, Casey A, Short A, Harris R, Soderlund K, Hultman E, "Influence of oral creatine supplementation on muscle torque during repeated bouts of maximal voluntary contraction in man," *Clin Sci* 84 (1993): 565-571.

Grindstaff P, Kreider R, Bishop R, Wilson M, Wood L, Alexander C, Almada A, "Effects of creatine supplementation on repetitive sprint performance and body composition in competitive swimmers," *Int J Sport Nutr* 7(4) (1997): 330-346.

Harris R, Viru M, Greenhaff P, Hultman E, "The effect of oral creatine supplementation on running performance during maximal short-term exercise in man," *J Physiol* 467 (1993): 74P, 1993.

Harris R, Soderlund K, Hultman E, "Elevation of creatine in resting and exercised muscles of normal subjects by creatine supplementation," *Clin Sci* 83 (1992): 367-374.

Haussinger D, Roth E, Lang F, Gerok W, "Cellular hydration state: an important determinant of protein catabolism in health and disease," *Lancet* 341 (1993): 1330-1332.

Hultman E, Soderlund K, Timmons J, Cederblad G, Greenhaff P, "Muscle creatine loading in men," *J Appl Physiol* 81(1) (1996): 232-237.

Kreider R, Ferreira M, Wilson M, Grindstaff P, Plisk S, Reinardy J, Cantler E, Almada A, "Effects of creatine supplementation on body composition, strength, and sprint performance," *Med Sci Sports Exerc* 30(1) (1998): 73-82.

Prevost M, Nelson A, Morris S, "Creatine supplementation enhances intermittent work performance," *Res Qrtly Exerc Sport* 68(3) (1997): 233-240.

Poortmans J, Auquier H, Renaut V, Durussel A, Saugy M, Brisson G, "Effect of short-term creatine supplementation on renal responses in men," *Eur J Appl Physiol* 76 (1997): 566-567.

Redondo D, Dowling E, Graham B, Alamada A, Williams M, "The effect of oral creatine monohydrate supplementation on running velocity," *Int J Sport Nutr* 6 (1996): 213-221.

Rossiter H, Cannell E, Jakeman P, "The effect of oral creatine supplementation on the 1,000-m performance of competitive rowers," *J Sports Sci* 14 (1996): 175-179.

Stockler S, Marescau B, De Deyn P, Trijbels J, Hanefeld F, "Guanidino compounds in guanidinoacetate methyltransferase deficiency, a new inborn error of creatine synthesis," *Metabolism* 46(10) (1997): 1189-1193.

Stroud M, Holliman D, Bell D, Green A, Macdonald I, Greenhaff P, "Effect of oral creatine supplementation on respiratory gas exchange and blood lactate accumulation during steady-state incremental treadmill exercise and recovery in man," *Clin Sci* 87 (1994): 707-710.

Tarnopolsky M, Roy B, MacDonald J, "A randomized, controlled trial of creatine monohydrate in patients with mitochondrial cytopathies," *Muscle Nerve* 20 (1997): 1502-1509.

Terrillion K, Kolkhorst F, Dolgener F, Joslyn S, "The effect of creatine supplementation on two 700-m maximal running bouts," *Int J Sport Nutr* 7(2) (1997): 138-143.

Thompson C, Kemp G, Sanderson A, Dixon R, Styles P, Taylor D, Radda G, "Effects of creatine on aerobic and anaerobic metabolism in skeletal muscle in swimmers," *Br J Sports Med* 30 (1996): 222-225.

Vandenberghe K, Gillis N, Van Leemputte M, Van Hecke P, Vanstapel F, Hespel P, "Caffeine counteracts the ergogenic action of muscle creatine loading," *J Appl Physiol* 80(2) (1996): 452-457.

Volek J, Kraemer W, Bush J, Boetes M, Incledon T, Clark K, Lynch J, "Creatine supplementation enhances muscular performance during high-intensity resistance exercise," *J Am Diet Assoc* 97 (1997): 765-770.

Waldegger S, Busch G, Kaba N, Zempel G, Ling H, Heidland A, Haussinger D, Lang F, "Effect of cellular hydration on protein metabolism," *Miner Electrolyte Metab* 23 (1997): 201-205.

Walker J, "Creatine biosynthesis, regulation and function," *Adv Enzymol* 50 (1979): 117-242.

Suggested Readings
and Resources

DiPasquale M. *Amino Acids and Proteins for the Athlete: The Anabolic Edge*. Boca Raton, FL: CRC Press, 1997.

Gastelu D and Hatfield F. *Dynamic Nutrition for Maximum Performance: A Complete Nutritional Guide for Peak Sports Performance*. Garden City Park, NY: Avery Publishing Group, 1997.

Kraemer W and Fleck S. *Designing Resistance Training Programs*, second edition. Champaign, IL: Human Kinetics, 1997.

Sahelian R and Tuttle D. *Creatine: Nature's Muscle Builder*. Garden City Park, NY: Avery Publishing Group, 1997.

Tuttle D. *Bigger, Faster, Stronger: 50 Ways to Build Muscle Fast*. Garden City Park, NY: Avery Publishing Group, 1998.

Web (Internet) Site
www. raysahelian.com

Index